Healthy Habits Books

# Coconut Oil

## 15 Highly Effective Healthy Habits That Help You Lose Weight FAST, Sleep Sound, Find Energy & Create Powerful and Effective Great Habits FOR LIFE

By Cathy Wilson

Copyright © 2015

Also, there are no resale rights or private label rights granted when purchasing this book. In other words, it's for your own personal use only.

Also, there are no resale rights or private label rights granted when purchasing this book. In other words, it's for your own personal use only.

# Coconut Oil

## 15 Highly Effective Healthy Habits That Help You Lose Weight FAST, Sleep Sound, Find Energy & Create Powerful and Effective Great Habits FOR LIFE

### I'm Not Perfect...But I'm REAL

*Please understand I can't yet afford a fancy-dancy publishing company to present my passionately written books perfectly - Not yet anyway! :)*

*TRANSLATION - Please don't blast me about the odd spelling error missed. Focus on what you gain.*

### My Knowledge is For You

*Perfect to me is when my fingers take over and dance across the keys. And if you gain just one piece of useful information from my creation, then I'm smiling!*

*Lastly, without reviews my books will not rank and they will not sell. That's important to me. I have 6 kids to feed! LOL- So, if you've a minute to spare and enjoyed my masterpiece, I'll be tickled rainbow if you left me a review. I'll even owe you one if you like!*

*Thanks for your time. Enjoy the show!*

*Cathy :)*

# Table of Contents

# Table of Contents

# Introduction

Undeniably coconut oil is one of nature's gifts that just keeps giving. The health benefits of this healthy saturated fat include better skin, improved hair and nails, weight loss, strengthened immune system function, better sleep, improved mood, healthier teeth, better digestion, and increased metabolism to burn fat faster.

*Sceptic nutritionist* says the benefits of coconut oil also include stress relief, reduction in kidney issues, decreased risk of heart disease, lower blood pressure, less risk of diabetes, HIV, cancer, and dental issues, and improved bone strength.

**The list of healthy benefits associated with coconut oil are endless!**

**COCONUT OIL FACTS**

1 tbsp. of coconut oil has 120 calories of saturate fat (13.6g fat) - made of rare HEALTHY medium chain triglycerides, according to coconutoil.com.

Studies report the link to weight loss and great health is with this configuration of the coconut oil fat fatty acid chain. Call it magic if you like, but the studies don't lie.

This saturated fat is the exception to rules for scientifically proven healthy saturated fat. A somewhat new world finding that's gaining positive momentum each day as researchers work tirelessly to uncover the deep medicinal secrets this all-natural healthy saturated fat contains.

I've personally experimented with this oil and have found only **POSITIVE** gain using it.

Time to find out more!

# Chapter One- 10 Coconut Oil Tips Weight Loss

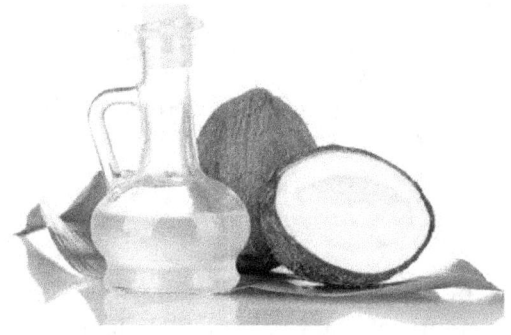

Coconut oil has all sorts of uses like managing your weight, controlling blood sugar, and boosting metabolism. Experts believe coconut oil used in moderation is valuable in setting you up for weight loss success.

Read on to find out more!

**Weight Loss Tip 1 - A Fat That Burns Fat!**

Research studies show coconut oil can remove inches from your waist while lowering your BMI. This is fantastic news! Keep in mind this doesn't mean you're going to lose weight. For that you've got to use more energy than you eat.

**GREAT NEWS** - Maybe what you eat can help you burn fat in all those tough places, like the belly area?

**Weight Loss Tip 2- Feel Fuller Longer**

Coconut oil is a saturated fat that helps appease your appetite longer. It fills you up and keeps you full longer than many other foods, especially simple sugar high calorie junk foods like chips, pastries, sweets, and white breads.

Experts also report this oil naturally slows down digestion.

Incorporating coconut oil into you day will encourage your body to eat less and feel more satisfied. That all adds up to **FAST** weight loss!

### Weight Loss Tip 3 - Control Blood Sugar

*WebMD* experts report coconut oil helps level blood sugars by providing constant rich energy longer. When you are "feeling" satisfied with what you ate you're less likely to binge on unhealthy high-fat sweet treats.

Coconut oil also levels cravings in studies. This gives you the chance to make better food choices and lose weight.

### Weight Loss Tip 4 - Readily Available Energy

Coconut oil provides pure energy that's ready to use. It's fast energy without the fat storage. *Coconutoiltips* reports your liver transforms the MCTs from coconut oil into energy that can be used immediately. No extra enzymes are required for the breakdown process.

This makes coconut oil a great option pre-workout!

### Weight Loss Tip 5 - Smooth's Out Cellulite

This one might not be weight loss directly, but I'm pretty sure you'd like to smooth out some of your fat for a more toned appearance! Research studies show when coconut oil is rubbed religious onto the skin for at least ten minutes per day, it may actually reduce the look of your bumpy fat.

I haven't tried this one yet but it's on my list!

**Weight Loss Tip 6 - Boost Metabolism**

Magic to your ears! *Authority Nutrition* experts state coconut oil is high in medium chain triglycerides, fatty acids that increase metabolism.

This specific type of fat metabolizes differently than longer chain fats. They go right to the liver and are used immediately or transformed into ketones.

Great news when you're looking to lose weight because a natural boost in metabolism means you're burning more calories so you can lose weight.

**Weight Loss Tip 7 - Start with a Tablespoon Each Day**

When looking to use coconut oil for weight loss you are best to just take it by the tablespoon. Start with just one tablespoon until your body gets used to it. Using it this way means you don't have to worry about losing any of the weight-blasting properties by overheating or somehow taking away its unique qualities.

Work your way up until you're taking 2-3 tablespoons daily for weight loss.

**Weight Loss Tip 8 - Balances Hormones**

If you aren't getting all of your fatty acids your body can't produce and regulate the hormones essential for things like digestion, sex, metabolism, and mood. The specialty fatty acids in coconut oil help your body convert cholesterol in your blood into pregnenolone (strerone).

**Translation** - Coconut oil specifically helps with hormone regulation, which in turn increases energy, reduces stress, improves digestion, and helps you lose weight!

**Weight Loss Tip 9 - Nutrient Absorption**

*Natural Living Ideas* experts report coconut oil may help your digestive tract better absorb fat-soluble vitamins (vitamins that need fat for absorption). Vitamins A, D, E, and K are essential for healthy skin, smooth brain function, better mood, and cell regeneration. When your system has all the vitamins it requires you feel better, look better, and naturally increase your odds at losing weight safely and effectively.

**Weight Loss Tip 10 - Commit to Regular**

If coconut oil is going to help in your plan to lose weight you've got to stick with it. This means taking your 2-3 tablespoons each day EVERY day. Skipping days or trying to take more or less isn't going to work.

It's all about balance and this is an instance where more isn't better!

Start off by setting yourself up to eat your daily dose of coconut oil for 30 days, and then start looking for results. For many it happens much sooner but the most important factor here is that you set up realistic expectations and set yourself up for long-term success!

*My Thoughts...*

*Coconut oil for weight loss seems to be the rave today. Keep in mind it will only work if you are using the oil in moderation,*

*combined with healthy eating, regular exercise, and a healthy lifestyle.*

*Permanent weight loss is a commitment for life. If you are willing to take action there's no doubt coconut oil can be a positive part of it!*

# Chapter Two - 10 Coconut Oil Tips for Skin and Hair

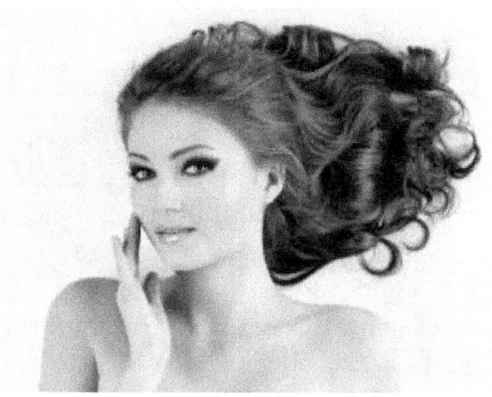

This is where my personal experiments come in. I've fooled around with virgin coconut oil and my skin and hair for about a year now, with impressive results. Studies show coconut oil has huge benefits for your hair and skin, and here are a few uncovered!

### Skin and Hair Tip 1 - Makeup Remover

*Readers Digest* reports coconut oil is perfect for removing stubborn makeup. All you do is dab a little onto a cotton ball and wipe to remove makeup. Be sure to rinse your face afterward because coconut oil can trigger breakouts if you are prone to oil skin.

### Skin and Hair Tip 2 - Repairs Damaged Split Ends - Tames Frizz

I don't need a research study to prove this one. My hair is naturally thin and straggly looking, always looking dry and unhealthy. By putting a tiny bit of coconut oil on the ends of my hair after regular shampoo and conditioner, I brought back life!

Be careful though cuz it doesn't take much to overdo it and turn your hair into a grease-ball.

**Skin and Hair Tip 3 - Deep Conditioner**

I recommend this especially if your hair is prone to oiliness. Just because your hair gets oil built up quickly doesn't mean it doesn't need conditioning. After you've washed your hair in the shower take about a tablespoon of coconut oil and massage it evenly through your hair. Leave on for 3-5 minutes and then rinse out thoroughly.

Your hair will look and feel amazing!

**Skin and Hair Tip 4 - Issues with Nails**

Coconut oil helps with anything from dryness around the nails, cuticle issues, minor nail infections, and even psoriasis. I've had minor bouts with all and after about 6 weeks of rubbing coconut oil directly onto my nails daily, my nail issues disappeared. In fact I believe my nails have strengthened.

My recommendation is to rub coconut oil onto your nails daily whether you have issues or not. It will only help make your nails beautiful!

**Skin and Hair Tip - 5 - Eczema**

My kids flare up with minor bouts of eczema. Usually it's just really dry skin but irritating and itchy nonetheless. I started rubbing coconut oil on the affected areas twice daily and within 2-3 weeks the dryness was completely gone. Now I'm not going to say it's gone forever. But the coconut oil definitely worked wonders to get rid of it this time around.

**Skin and Hair Tip - 6 - Wrinkles Be Gone!**

Here's another one I've personally put to the test. Each night before bed I apply a small amount of coconut oil around my eyes, forehead, and around my mouth. After about a month I noticed an overall improvement in my skin in these areas. It felt firmer and definitely looked healthier.

Why didn't I put it all over my face?

I have combination skin and tend to break out if I put the oil all over.

**Skin and Hair Tip - 7 - Deodorant**

*RD.com* reports coconut oil has a bacteria called lauric acid that kills odor. All you've got to do is dab a little under your armpits to stay fresh and dry all day. Haven't tried this one but I will!

**Skin and Hair Tip - 8 - Bath Moisturizer**

I LOVE using coconut oil in and after my bath for smooth healthy looking skin. I usually put 2 tablespoons in my bath, and apply as a body moisturizer after I get out. It doesn't take much to make your skin soft and beautiful.

As you are rubbing it in the heat from your body will turn it into liquid quickly. Just keep rubbing it in till your skin soaks it all up. Rub off excess with a towel if you have to.

**Skin and Hair Tip - 9 - Lip Balm**

Here's another one I use daily. Just dab a little coconut oil on your lips and rub it in with your finger. This helps moisturize and protect you lips from the harsh elements of nature.

If you like you can put a little in a small container to put in your purse or pocket. It's handy and works awesome.

**Skin and Hair Tip - 10 - Cold Sores Go Away**

Research studies show that dabbing a touch of coconut oil onto a cold sore as it develops helps to speed up the healing process. It's the medicinal antiviral properties of the oil that takes action. And this is one instance where more is better.

*My Thoughts...*

*Coconut oil has a zillion uses and my suggestion to you is just test it out for yourself. You'll be surprised how much healing power this all-natural oil has. The key is to be persistent. If you are using it to treat minor skin ailments you've gotta give it a chance to work.*

# Chapter Three- Myth or Truth?

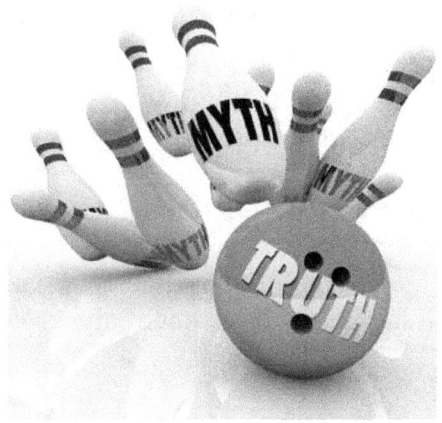

*Health Impact News* comes in handy when it comes to battling coconut oil rumors with inaccurate information. They report that coconut oil has been around for centuries and researched extensively for over 15 years. So when you read something talking about how coconut oil is a "fad" or "all hype," then you're reading Myth 1 and 2!

**Here are a few myths that need debunking!**

**Myth 1 - Stay away from coconut oil because it causes heart disease!**

**TRUTH -** Loads of epidemiological studies have been done for years and saturate fat has never been PROVEN to cause cardiovascular disease.

Look into the Ketogenic Diet for a better understanding. This high-fat diet was created by doctors to help treat and cure epilepsy in children where drug therapy wasn't effective.

Unfortunately this myth about saturated fat (coconut oil) causing heart disease scared people off from using the Ketogenic Diet to help children battling epilepsy.

Luckily in recent years the tables have turned and the benefits of coconut oil are widespread. Helping all sorts of conditions from epilepsy and dementia, to Alzheimer's and cancer.

**Myth 2 - I'm allergic to coconut oil, so I can't eat it.**

**TRUTH -** This one is HIGHLY unlikely. In most cases it's not an allergy to coconut oil, but an issue with the intestine function of fat. Perhaps the inability to digest various types of protein. So the issue is more likely with the protein and not the oil.

You can try and desensitize yourself to coconut oil if you having issues with digestion and experiencing symptoms like diarrhea, bloating, gas and skin issues. To do this just reduce the amount of coconut oil to eat to smaller amounts. Continue this until the symptoms lessen and disappear. Then you should be able to enjoy coconut oil without issue.

**Myth 3 - Coconut oil is sweet and bad for diabetics.**

**TRUTH -** Coconut oil is definitely not sweet tasting. According to *WEB MD* coconut oil is pure fat and has no glucose in it. Add to that coconut oil actually helps with diabetes because it encourages the release of insulin from the pancreas, which helps control diabetes.

**Myth 4 - Coconut oil tastes yucky.**

**TRUTH -** That's totally subjective, so it's not true. Coconut oil solo may not appeal to you, but when you use it for cooking or baking, I bet you're singing a different tune. Same as tomatoes for some people. You may not like tomatoes but how about tomato sauce or ketchup?

To each his/her own with this one.

**Myth 5 - All coconut oil has a high smoke point for cooking.**

**TRUTH -** *The Nutrition Guru and the Chef* Health experts set the record straight with this one. NOT ALL Coconut oil has a high smoke point (meaning you can heat it hotter before the chemical structures is altered or damaged and may produce carcinogens).

Only REFINED coconut oil has the stabilizers added to increase the smoke point. And the most common virgin cold pressed coconut oil actually has a very low smoke point compared to other oils. This means it shouldn't be used on high heat.

For cooking you are best to look for macadamia or grape seed oil, with higher smoke points.

*My Thoughts...*

*With so much information readily available there's bound to be some wires crossed. If something doesn't make sense to you make sure you investigate further to get to the truth. You can do some research on your own, speak with your doctor, or another health professional that will give you the nuts and bolts facts of the matter.*

At least with the truth you can create a solid plan to reach your healthy goals FAST!

# Chapter Four- 5 Surprise Uses for Coconut Oil

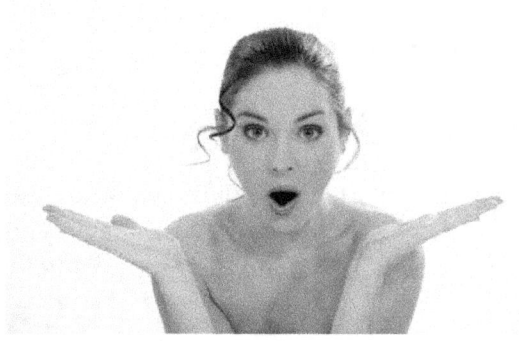

### Surprise Use 1 - Head Lice

Experts suggest soaking the infected heat in apple cider vinegar to dry. Then apply coconut oil into the hair and leave on overnight. This gives the oil time to smother and kill the lice.

Afterward wash as usual and comb through the hair with lice comb.

### Surprise Use 2 - Protect Minor Wounds

*Woman's Day* reports rubbing a small amount of coconut oil on minor wounds after they've been cleaned helps to keep away bacteria or dust. A fast and easy way to keep infection away.

### Surprise Use 3 - Cradle Cap

_Naturalnews.com_ experts recommend using coconut oil to get handle on newborn cradle cap. There's nothing dangerous about cradle cap, but it is annoying. A yellowish scaling of the skin while your baby is adjusting from a wet to dry environment.

Just rub a dollop of coconut oil on the affected area 2-3 times per day and notice immediate improvement.

**Surprise Use 4 - Baby Thrush**

Check with your doctor first, but many health experts recommend applying a small dab of coconut oil inside your baby's mouth on the affected area and on the nipple to help prevent infection.

The natural antifungal properties of coconut oil help with this issues.

**Surprise Use 5 - Sunscreen**

According to _Chatelaine Magazine_ coconut oil acts as a mild skin protectant with a natural SPF of 7. So it's not enough to completely protect you from the sun's rays but it does help. Use it to nourish your skin before and after sun for added benefits.

_My Thoughts..._

_If you dig deep enough you can find some really powerful and unusual uses for coconut oil. Nothing surprises me when it comes to the health benefits of using coconut oil in your day._

# Chapter Five- Science of Coconut Oil

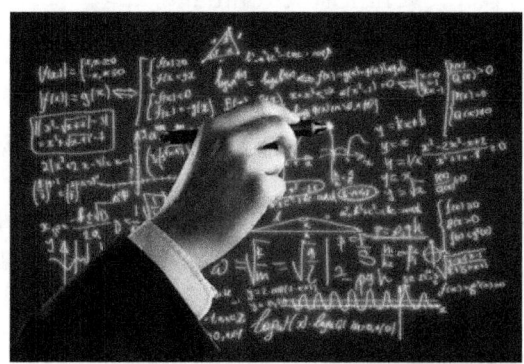

Many people need the scientific evidence before they'll consider anything fact. Science isn't the end all be all of truth. But it certainly does help validate some of the health benefit claims of this seemingly miraculous natural oil.

May the truth be told through science!

**COCONUT OIL FACTS WITH SCIENCE TO BACK THEM...**

### Heart Disease

*The Department of Human Biology, University of Maastricht* states recent research shows all saturated fats don't trigger cardiovascular disease. Research shows pure coconut oil lowers LDL (bad) cholesterol and increases HDL (good) cholesterol levels. This naturally lowers your risk of heart disease.

### Healthy Hair

Studies show coconut oil treats damaged hair by infiltrating into the damaged ends and moisturizing. It helps reduce protein loss and the lauric acid in the oil has an affinity for hair proteins since it has a low weight it penetrates through to the hair fibers and helps prevent further damage.

## Immune Function

According to studies from the *Payap University, Thailand,* the lauric acid found in coconut oil increases your body's output of monolaurin, which improves antibacterial protection. It's also well known that coconut oil has natural analgesic and anti-inflammatory abilities to further ward off disease and illness.

## Treatment Alzheimer's

*Dr. Mary Newport* has discovered numerous benefits using coconut oil to treat Alzheimer's. Studies have found a portion of this disease may be "diabetes of the brain." Where the brain isn't taking in enough glucose function. This takes 10 to 20 years to develop. The good news is ketones can replace the glucose needed for brain function.

The ketones from coconut oil in particular prove especially receptive for Alzheimer's treatment.

## South Pacific Cultures Disease-Free

Coconutdiet.com reports a study conducted on 2 South Pacific populations at times before unhealthy western foods were introduced, found people were very healthy with very little modern disease. Back ten these people consumed up to 60% of their diet from coconuts.

*POINTER* - It's the "type" of saturated fat that causes health issues.

## Skin Health

Research studies from the *Department of Dermatology, Philippines,* show coconut oil improves atopic dermatitis by moisturizing. This oil can also be used to aid with minor cuts and burns, and relieves moderate xerosis.

**Athletic Performance Enhancement**

Scientific studies show the MCTs from coconut oil are quickly digested into the bloodstream, so they can be used for fast energy. The result is increased athletic performance.

*My Thoughts...*

*Science says coconut oil has huge health benefits in pretty much all aspects of health. From improving your natural glow, to preventing disease and promoting weight loss, coconut oil has something to say.*

*Like it or lump it, you're wise-owl smart to be experimenting with coconut oil in your life!*

# Final Thoughts...

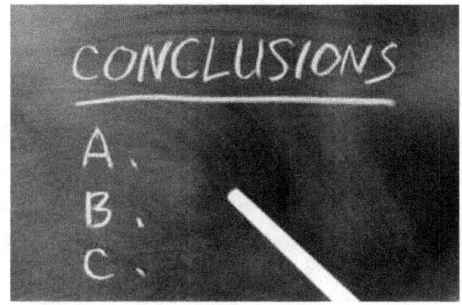

*Organicfacts.net* says according to the *Coconut Research Center*, coconut oil...

*Kills the viruses that cause the flu, herpes, measles, hepatitis, and other serious disease
*Kills bacteria that causes breathing issues, pneumonia, throat infections, ulcers, bladder infections, and gonorrhea
*Eliminates the fungi that triggers yeast causing athlete's food, diaper rash, thrush, yeast infection and ringworm

**Add to this...**

*Dissolving kidney stones
*Preventing liver disease
*Eliminating stress
*Preventing and treating diabetes
*Improving dental hygiene
*Strengthening bones
*Deterring cancer and HIV
*Boosting immune system function

*Treating Alzheimer's
*Boosting metabolism
*Blasting fat
*Improving mood
*Increasing energy
*Reducing the signs of aging
*Strengthening hair
*Healing wounds
*Relieving minor skin irritations
*Improving digestion
*Balances hormones
*Deter heart disease

**What more do you want?**

You've got all the take-action information you need to lose weight, sleep better, gain energy, and improve your overall health and wellness immensely.

**All that's left for you to do is apply!**

# BONUS CHAPTER - 15 Highly Effective Healthy Habits That Help You Lose Weight FAST, Sleep Sound, Find Energy & Create Powerful and Effective Great Habits FOR LIFE!

**Healthy Habit 1 - Oil Pulling**

*Foodmatters.tv* reports numerous studies show oil pulling by swishing coconut oil around in your mouth 10-15 minutes each night will improve you overall oral health. This helps remove germs, bacteria and plaque, along with strengthening gums, teeth, and jaws.

**Healthy Habit 2 - Skin Scrub**

Skin experts recommend regular exfoliation for healthy younger looking skin. By combining equal parts coconut oil to sea salt, you've created an excellent facial scrub that sloughs off dead skin and deeply moisturizes.

Careful not to overdo it. 2-3 times a week is plenty.

**Healthy Habit 3 - Shaving Cream**

A healthy skin habit is using coconut oil as shaving cream. The coconut oil works well as a lubricant and moisturizer, particularly good for sensitive skin.

**Healthy Habit 4 - Cure Insomnia**

*Thevirgincoconutoil.com* reports coconut oil may cure insomnia. Coconut oil has the ability to help level hormones and system internal function. This helps your body settle down for a solid sleep without interference.

Add to this...

*10-15 minutes sun exposure every day
*Calming bedtime ritual with NO stimulants (exercising, caffeine, bright lights, loud music, electronics)

**Healthy Habit 5 - Fat Loss**

Coconut oil has been proven time and again to aid in weight loss. The medium chain fatty acids aid in burning fat and smooth digestion. This oil also helps improve the function of the endocrine and thyroid systems, according to organicfacts.net. Stress is also taken off the pancreas which boosts metabolism for increased energy burn.

Just look to the tropical coastal areas where coconut oil is a staple. You'll find very little disease or obese people.

**Healthy Habit 6 - Pancreas**

Prevention: Coconut oil has proven helpful in treating pancreatitis.

**Healthy Habit 7 - Bones Health**

Studies show coconut oil helps with the absorption of vitamins and minerals. Which includes calcium essential decreasing the risk of osteoporosis. This is especially important for women entering menopause and beyond.

**Healthy Habit 8 - Cancer and HIV**

Creating a healthy habit of taking 2-3 tablespoons of coconut oil each day will help reduce chances of infection, stemming from HIV and cancer, according to studies conducted by *Cancer Research of America.*

## Healthy Habit 9 - Coconut Oil and Bee Pollen

*Entrepreneur.com* reports eating a teaspoon of bee pollen with a drizzle of coconut oil provides instant energy to last the day! The bee pollen is providing lots of benefits and is loaded with vital nutrients that help with stamina and focus.

The MCTs in coconut oil speed up your metabolism and blast fact. The perfect combination!

## Healthy Habit 10 - Lift Mood

Adding a tablespoon of pure coconut oil to your morning smoothie will put the zip into your step pronto! I usually have a Blueberry Banana Spinach Smoothie for breakfast. And when I want a touch more energy I just toss in a spoonful of coconut oil. YUMMY!

Ingredients:

1 large banana
1/2 cup yogurt
1/2 cup ice
1 cup spinach
1/2 cup blueberries
1/2 cup milk
1 tbsp. coconut oil

Blend!

**Healthy Habit 11 - Cook With Coconut Oil**

Instead of buttering or greasing up you stir-fry pan, use a table-spoon of coconut oil instead. The oil adds good fat, protective medicine, and succulent flavor to your dishes.

Just remember moderation is critical. Don't overdo it or you WILL eventually gain weight!

**Healthy Habit 12 - Hand/Foot Treatment**

If you a looking to indulge and give your hands and feet a makeover, start by lathering them up in coconut oil and putting on a pair of old pair of gloves and socks for the night. The cotton will allow for breathing and enable you natural body heat to open pores and allow for deep absorption.

Come morning time your feet and hand will be nourished and silky soft smooth!

**Healthy Habit 13 - Massaging**

Here's another healthy habit you're going to need to get your partner to take charge of. Not only is a massage with coconut oil beneficial for relaxation and de-stressing, but it also helps provide the much needed moisture most skin lacks. Your skin vibrancy will come back and aches and pains will disappear.

**Healthy Habit 14 - Roasted Veggies in Coconut Oil for Weight Loss**

When you're roasting up those fresh veggies for dinner make sure you're using a dollop of coconut oil instead of your usual butter or veggie oil. The coconut oil adds a tasty flavor and aroma, along with the healthy fat you need to lose weight FAST, according to *Shape Magazine.*

**Healthy Habit 15 - COMMIT!**

The healthiest most important move you can make is to COMMIT to getting 2-3 tablespoons of coconut oil into your day instead of other unhealthy saturated fats. Keep everything in moderation and make sure you start using this medicinal oil to make you skin and hair beautiful, clear up minor wounds and skin conditions, and you can even use it to take off makeup and starve off lice.

**Coconut oil can will reach out and touch your life positively if you let it!**

*Last Thoughts…*

**\*THANK-YOU** for reading my masterpiece. I hope you learned a little something, or at least got a few smiles.
\*I would appreciate a millisecond or three of your time for a quick review, to help me build my masterful book empire higher.
\*Whatever you do, don't forget to smile, and of course, check out my website for more of my e-Book masterpieces at: www.flawlesscreativewriting.com

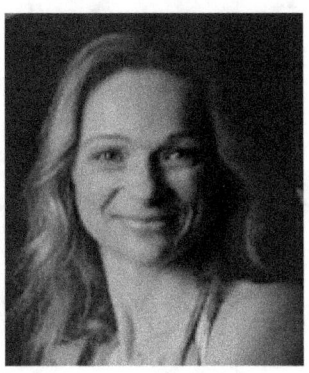

Cathy☺

Disclaimer